Copyright © 2020 Laura Summers

All rights reserved. No part of this publication

may be reproduced, distributed, or transmitted

in any form or by any means, including

photocopying, recording, or other electronic or

mechanical methods, without the prior written

permission of the publisher, except in the case

of brief quotations embodied in critical reviews

and certain other noncommercial uses

permitted by copyright law.

Table of Contents

INTRODUCTION

An autoimmune disease causes the immune system to attack and damage healthy tissues or organs by mistake.

Common examples of this type of disease include psoriasis, rheumatoid arthritis, and lupus.

An autoimmune disease can cause inflammation, and fatigue is another common symptom. Depending on the condition, additional symptoms may include pain, swelling, skin changes, and a fever.

The AIP diet may help reduce inflammation and other symptoms of autoimmune conditions. Learn more about the diet and its potential effects below.

How to follow the AIP diet

A person on the AIP diet can eat most vegetables.

The AIP is an elimination diet, so it involves not eating certain types of food for several weeks at a time and carefully noting any effects on health. Researchers have described the AIP diet as an extension of the paleo diet. A person usually eats lean proteins, vegetables, fruits, nuts, and seeds. The AIP diet focuses on foods rich in vitamins and other nutrients. A person following it will not eat anything with added sugar or other additives that can trigger an autoimmune response. A person should adhere to the diet strictly for a few weeks, then slowly reintroduce the eliminated foods and take careful note of any reaction. A reaction, such as a surge in symptoms, can indicate that they should exclude that food in the long term.

Foods to eat and avoid

Foods to eat

Limited research indicates which specific foods the AIP diet includes. A person following the diet may be able to eat:

- any vegetables, except those from the nightshade family

- high-quality seafood that are rich in omega-3 fatty acids

- fermented foods

- lean meats and liver

- small amounts of fruit

- oils, such as olive, coconut, and avocado oils

In general, the diet focuses on whole foods and those that do not contain additives such as sugar.

Foods to avoid

There are several food groups to avoid when following an AIP diet.Little guidance is tailored to people with any specific autoimmune condition, but a study in people with IBS recommends avoiding:

- nightshades, such as tomatoes, potatoes, peppers, and eggplants

- grains

- legumes

- dairy

- some vegetable oils

- coffee

- eggs

- nuts and seeds

- alcohol

- food additives, such as refined or added sugars.

One day AIP Diet Plan

Below are examples of meals that you could eat on the AIP diet:

Breakfast

- Organic bacon
- Sweet potato

Lunch

- Sautéed kale, and zucchini
- Chicken and ginger stir-fry
- Cauliflower rice

Dinner

- Roasted cauliflower and pumpkin soup

- Zucchini noodles with salmon and basil pesto

Snacks

- Smoothies

- "nice cream" (frozen banana and coconut milk ice cream)

- Coconut yoghurt and berries

- Carob cookies

RECIPES

Hydrating Berry Popsicles

Prep time: 12 hours

Serving: 12

Ingredients

- 1 1/2 cups Blackberries

- 1 1/2 cups Blueberries

- 3 cups Strawberries

- 3 cups Coconut Water, unsweetened

- 2 Tablespoon Raw Honey

Process

1. Place the blackberries, one cup of coconut water, and two teaspoons of

honey into a blender. Blend until smooth.

2. Strain the mixture through a fine mesh strainer to remove the blackberry seeds, and set aside.

3. Repeat this process two more times with the strawberries and blueberries, using 1 cup of coconut water per flavor of berry, and 2 teaspoons of honey.

4. Be sure that all three flavors are strained into separate bowls.

5. Pour the blueberries in the first 3rd of your popsicle molds, and freeze until solid.

6. Repeat with the strawberries and blackberries.

7. Once you have filled the last flavor into your molds, freeze overnight, or for at least 6 hours.

Notes

We have a popsicle mold that uses loose sticks, and they are secured in place by the lid to the mold. When the strawberry layer was mostly frozen, I removed the lid, and just let the sticks sit in the mostly frozen mixture so that I would be able to fill the final layer with the sticks in place. This was a bit tricky, but worked fine in the end.

Summer Pasta(less) Salad

This is based off of a spaghetti salad my mom made when I was growing up. The first time I made the paleo version, I prepped myself before I took the first bite to remind myself it wouldn't be quite as good. I was very wrong! I loved the crisp noodles and flavors of the vegetables so much more than a wheat-based noodle. This is a great side dish to bring to a summer barbecue or party!

Prep time: 25 minutes

Cook time: 25 minutes

Servings: 8

Ingredients

- 2 1/2 lb Yellow Squash (peeled and spiralized into noodles)
- 1/2 cup Green Onion (sliced)
- 1/2 whole Cucumber (quartered and sliced)
- 6 oz Black Olives
- 1/2 cup Extra Virgin Olive Oil, (for the dressing)
- 3 tablespoons Apple Cider Vinegar, (for the dressing)
- 1/2 tablespoon Garlic Powder, (for the dressing)
- 3/4 tablespoon Onion Powder, (for the dressing)

- 1 1/2 tablespoon dried Oregano, (for the dressing)

(caution: the strictest form of AIP eliminates black pepper, leave it out if you are sensitive)NaN

- 1/8 tablespoon Thyme, (for the dressing)
- 1/2 tablespoon dried Basil, (for the dressing)
- 3/4 tablespoon Parsley, (for the dressing)
- 3/4 tablespoon Sea Salt, (for the dressing)

Process

1. Place all veggies in a large bowl.

2. Place all dressing ingredients in a small glass jar. Shake in mix thoroughly.

3. Pour dressing over veggies and toss to combine.

4. Serve cold.

Pan Roasted Pork Chops (AIP-friendly)

This is a super-flavorful way to prepare pork chops which avoids the common pitfalls of being bland or dry. You're going to LOVE this recipe!

Prep time: 10 minutes

Cook time: 20 minutes

Servings: 2

Ingredients

- 1 1/2 lb Pork Chop, two chops, about 3/4 lb each, bone in.
- 1 Tablespoon Primal Palate Super Gyro Seasoning

- 2 Tablespoons Lard, or your choice of cooking fat. We also really like Primal Kitchen Avocado Oil.

- 2 Tablespoons Tin Star Cultured Ghee

- 2 cloves Garlic, crushed

- fresh Thyme, a few sprigs

- 1/4 Tablespoon Sea Salt, to garnish

Process

1. Bring the pork chops out 15-20 minutes prior to cooking to allow to come up to room temperature.

2. Sprinkle Super Gyro seasoning on all sides, and allow the chops to rest.

3. Preheat your oven to 425 F.

4. In a medium cast iron skillet, heat 2 tablespoons of cooking fat over medium heat. (The new Primal Kitchen Avocado Oil is awesome for this, but you can also use Lard or Coconut Oil.) When the oil starts to shimmer, tilt the pan to evenly coat it with the oil, and add the pork chops.

5. Sear on the first side for 3:30, then flip and sear the second side for 3 minutes. Flip again for 2 minutes, and then a final time for 2 minutes. This helps to ensure an even sear.

6. Transfer the skillet to the hot oven. Flip the pork chops every 2 minutes, for a total of 10 minutes of roasting.

7. Remove the skillet from the oven. Move the pork chops to a plate, and drain off the fat from the skillet. Add 2 tablespoons of cultured ghee to the pan over medium heat. Add the crushed garlic and thyme to the pan, and saute for a minute.

8. Move the pork chops back to the hot pan, and spoon the ghee, thyme, and garlic over the chops. Cook for a final minute, continuing to spoon the ghee over the chops, and then remove to serve.

9. Allow the pork chops to rest a few minutes, then sprinkle with a moderately coarse sea salt (Like our

French Grey Sea Salt). Serve hot with your choice of side dishes!

"Super Gyro" Roasted Chicken Thighs

Prep time: 5 minutes

Cook time: 1 hour and 10 minutes

Servings: 2

Ingredients

- 1 Tablespoon Avocado Oil

- 12 cloves Garlic, (a fist, unpeeled)

- 4 skin on Chicken Thigh

- 1 Tablespoon Primal Palate Super Gyro Seasoning

- pinch Himalayan Pink Salt

Process

1. Preheat your oven to 350 F.

2. Heat a medium pot over medium heat with the avocado oil, and saute the garlic cloves for 2-3 minutes (until the skins begin to brown.

3. In a large skillet over medium high heat, sear the chicken thighs on both sides (do skin-side first so they do not stick) - about 2-3 minutes per side.

4. Place the chicken over the garlic, and season with salt and Primal Palate Super Gyro blend.

5. Bake for an hour, covered. Serve along side your choice of vegetable.

Weeknight Roasted Chicken & Veggies

This recipe is part of my "I'm only human" recipe collection as it's easy enough to make on a weeknight. Use frozen vegetables like sweet potato and broccoli (or whatever you have on hand!) to minimize prep work. Be sure to use a chicken around 3.5 pounds so it cooks quickly.

Prep time: 10 minutes

Cook time: 1 hour and 15 minutes

Servings: 4

Ingredients

- 1 lb Sweet Potato, frozen and cubed, or sub another starchy vegetable

- 2 Tablespoons Extra Virgin Olive Oil, divided

- 7/8 Tablespoon Salt, divided

- 2 3/4 Tablespoon Primal Palate Garlic & Herb Seasoning, divided, or sub your favorite seasoning blend

- 1 lb Broccoli, florets, or sub other vegetable

- 3 1/2 lb Whole Chicken

Process

1. Preheat oven to 425°F.

2. Toss sweet potatoes in 1 Tablespoons olive oil with about 1/4 Tablespoon salt and 1/2 Tablespoon seasoning blend (or just season to taste!). Place in the bottom of a roasting pan.

3. Season the broccoli with about 1/8 Tablespoon salt and 1/4 Tablespoon of the seasoning blend (once again, you can just season to taste if you like). Add this to the roasting pan with the sweet potatoes.

4. Rinse the chicken, if desired, and pat dry with a paper towel. Rub the skin with 1 Tablespoons olive oil and about 1/2 Tablespoon salt and 2 Tablespoon seasoning blend.

5. Secure the legs and wings to the chicken with kitchen twine and place in the middle of the roasting dish. Breast-up, breast-down... I know everyone argues about that so I'll leave it up to you. I did mine breast-up so if you do-breast down, it may cook differently. You may want to scoot the vegetables out from under the chicken to around the edges of the pan.

6. Cover the roasting pan with foil and bake for 45 minutes. This prevents the spices from burning. After 45 minutes, remove the foil and continue baking until the temperature of the chicken reaches 165°F. You can check for

doneness by inserting a meat thermometer into the meatiest part of the inner thigh but make sure it's not touching bone. It will likely take another 20-30 minutes to fully cook after removing the foil.

Mashed Cauliflower Breakfast Bowls

These Mashed Cauliflower Breakfast Bowls are perfect for anyone needing a break from their typical breakfast smoothie or bacon and egg routine. While it's definitely a healthy AIP and gluten free recipe, it also has tons of flavor. The recipe is low carb, AIP & Whole 30 friendly, dairy free, and high in antioxidants. Regardless of the diet you're following, this breakfast bowl has you covered.

Prep time: 10 minutes

Cook time: 20 minutes

Servings: 2

Ingredients

- 1 whole Cauliflower

- 1 1/2 cup Baby Bella Mushrooms, or one 6 oz package

- 4 cup Arugula

- 6 pieces Bacon

- 1/4 cup Coconut Milk, you'll add this 1 Tablespoons at a time, and may not use it all

- 3 Tablespoons Coconut Aminos

- 1 Tablespoons Beef, Great Lakes brand Unflavored Gelatin

- 1 Tablespoons Nutritional Yeast

- 2 Tablespoons Bacon Grease, I suggest reserving grease from cooking the bacon, but you can also use ghee, coconut oil, or avocado oil

- 1 Tablespoons Extra Virgin Olive Oil

- 2 Tablespoon Sea Salt, or season to taste

Process

FOR THE MASHED CAULIFLOWER

1. Start by removing the leafy part of the stem, and roughly chop the head of cauliflower. It's okay to include the rest of the stem since the cauliflower will be steamed and blended.

2. Steam chopped cauliflower using your method of choice. I recommend a stovetop method.

3. Add steamed cauliflower to a blender or food processor. You can also do this with an immersion blender or by hand, but I find the blender and food processor to be the simplest and tends to yield the best consistency.

4. Add nutritional yeast (optional to provide a cheesy flavor), gelatin (to provide a thicker texture), about 1-2 Tablespoon sea salt, and 1 Tablespoons coconut milk. You'll want to start with just 1 Tablespoons coconut milk, but you'll likely need more depending on how much moisture is retained in your cauliflower.

5. Blend until smooth. Increase coconut milk by the tablespoon until desired consistency is reached. Be sure to test cauliflower to make sure it's salted to your liking.

FOR THE MUSHROOMS

1. Heat oil in a sauté pan over medium low heat.

1. Slice mushrooms in half and add to sauté pan. Cook slowly over low heat for the flavors to fully develop.

2. When the mushrooms are well cooked, pour in the Coconut Aminos to deglaze the pan and develop a caramelization on the outside of the mushrooms.

3. Remove from heat and sprinkle with a
   bit of coarse sea salt while the glaze is
   still wet.

FOR THE BACON

1. Preheat oven to 375 degrees.

2. Lay bacon on a rimmed, parchment
   lined baking sheet. Cook until crisp,
   about 12-15 minutes.

3. Remove bacon from cooking sheet and
   set aside to cool on a paper towel. This
   will absorb extra grease. Reserve the
   grease left on the baking sheet and
   store in an airtight jar in the fridge to
   use for cooking.

4. Once bacon has cooled, rough chop and
   store until use.

ASSEMBLY

1. Divide ingredients among 2 bowls, and
   drizzle with olive or avocado oil.
   Sprinkle with coarse sea salt.

2. These ingredients can be prepped the
   day before and reheated for a quick
   breakfast bowl, or eaten straight from
   the fridge

Delicata Squash Super Gyro Sliders

Prep time: 5 minutes

Cook time: 45 minutes

Servings: 8

Ingredients

- 2 lb Ground Beef, grass fed, 85% lean

- 2 whole Delicata Squash

- 1 Tablespoons Primal Palate Super Gyro Seasoning

- 5 pieces Bacon

- 1 whole Avocado

- 4 sprig Cilantro

- 1 whole Lime

- 1/2 Tablespoon Himalayan Pink Salt

Process

1. Pre-heat oven to 400F.

2. Place your bacon strips flat on the sheet pan and place in the cold oven while it pre-heats.

3. Cook bacon here for 10-15 minutes, until crispy.

4. Remove from the oven when done to your liking. Do not turn oven off.

5. Drain some of the fat off the sheet pan into a ramekin, set aside. Leave about 2 Tablespoons on the sheet pan.

6. Slice your delicate squash into 1/2 inch rings. Use a spoon to remove the seeds.

7. Place your rings on the greased sheet pan and flip over to grease both sides of

the rings with bacon fat. Sprinkle lightly with salt, about 1/4 Tablespoon, save the rest.

8. Place the squash in the oven. Bake for 15 minutes. Then gently flip the rings over. Bake another 5 minutes, or until fork tender.

9. In the meantime, in a large bowl mix the ground beef, seasoning, salt and bacon fat. Shape 6-8 sliders.

10. Remove the squash from the oven. Use a spatula to remove the squash from the sheet pan, set aside.

11. Arrange burger sliders on the sheet pan and roast at 400F for 15 minutes.

12. When they are done, place a slider over each ring.

13. Peel your avocado and smash it. Spoon a littler over each patty.

14. Sprinkle a little salt over them, then a little lime juice. Top with a few cilantro leaves.

15. Lastly, cut up the bacon in to 1/2 inch chunks and top your sliders off.

16. Viola! Delectable, seasonal, satisfying!

AIP Banana Mug Cake

Prep time: 2 minutes

Cook time: 3 minutes

Servings: 1

Ingredients

- 1 whole Banana, peeled

- 1 Tablespoons Organic Coconut Oil, solid, not melted

- 2 Tablespoons Coconut Milk

- 1/2 Tablespoon Pure Vanilla Extract

- 2 Tablespoons Coconut Flour

- 1 Tablespoon ground Cinnamon

- 1/4 Tablespoon Baking Soda

Process

1. Mash the banana and add the coconut oil, coconut milk, and vanilla.

2. Add the coconut flour, cinnamon, and baking soda; mix well.

3. Transfer to a ramekin or coffee cup.

4. Microwave on HIGH (100 percent power) for 3 minutes.

5. Cool a bit and enjoy.

Anti-Inflammatory Turmeric Tea

This recipe will be your best frand during cold and flu season. Personally I think this tea tastes amazing. And I am not a tea drinker. My idea of tea used to be McDonald's Sweet Tea... yeah, I've moved on to bigger an better things these days. Not to mention this tea is a combination of things that will do a body good. I mean GOOD. Let me break it down for you:

Turmeric: This spice is a member of the ginger root family, and is known for its anti-inflammatory effects. In fact, in India, it is widely used for arthritis and joint pain relief. A main compound of turmeric, curcumin, has been shown in at least 30 different studies to have anti-tumor/anticancer and antioxidant effects. This spice has also been shown to be a wonderful detoxing agent for the liver. Ginger: A classic for settling an upset stomach, this root too has anti-inflammatory effects. Ginger has also been shown to improve circulation, and has been used in Asian cultures for hundreds of years to treat cold hands and feet. Cinnamon: Cinnamon has been shown to lower blood sugar by increasing glucose metabolism, and also to improve capillary function. This spice also has antimicrobial and anti-inflammatory effects.

Prep time: 2 minutes

Cook time: 10 minutes

Servings: 1

Ingredients

- 1 cup Water

- 1/4 Tablespoon Turmeric Powder

- 1/4 Tablespoon ground Cinnamon

- 1/4 Tablespoon ground Ginger

- 1/2 Tablespoon Raw Honey

- 1 Tablespoons Lemon Juice

Process

1. In a small saucepan, bring the water to a steam (not quite to a boil, the hotter it gets, the longer you have to wait for it to cool.)

2. Add the spices, honey and lemon juice, and stir to combine.

3. Remove the saucepan from heat, and cover with a lid.

4. Allow the mixture to steam and combine for 10 minutes.

5. Drink once cooled. This tea will settle as you drink it, so you will need a spoon to redistribute the spices.

Autoimmune-Friendly Pumpkin Spice Cake w/ Gingersnap Crust

I am so thrilled to share with you the best holiday recipe I have come up with this year – Pumpkin Spice Cake with Gingersnap Crust! , I think that everyone needs a compliant dessert recipe they can share with their family and friends during the holidays. Since I have stopped eating sugar, I find that I am very sensitive to it, so in the development of this recipe my family and friends got to eat a lot of cake. A couple of tips before you get started: Arrowroot powder is much cheaper if you can find it in 20oz bags instead of the little jars they sell in the spice department. You can purchase online here, or ask for it at your local grocery. Next, you can make the cake with fresh roasted pumpkin or the canned variety, just make sure that the cans are BPA-free and have no other ingredients (like thickeners or spices). To cook the pumpkin, slice in half, remove the seeds, and cook for 60-90 minutes at 400 degrees. I find that a 2 1/2 pound pie pumpkin yields about 3 cups of puree. Lastly, the secret ingredient here, instead of coconut is lard. I recommend rendering your own, from a pastured source of leaf lard – here is a tutorial if you have never done it before. I have made this cake using both coconut oil and lard, and it tastes good both ways – but my family and I both prefer the lard version. Enjoy, and

please let me know if this allergy-friendly cake
is a hit.

Prep time: 30 minutes

Cook time: 30 minutes

Servings: 7

Ingredients

1. 3/4 cup Arrowroot Powder, + 1/3 cup

2. 1/4 Tablespoon Sea Salt, + 1/4
   Tablespoon

3. 1 1/2 cups Dates (Medjool), pitted and
   soaked in hot water for 5 minutes

4. 1 1/2 Tablespoon Ginger Root, grated

5. 3 cups Pumpkin Puree

6. 1/2 cup Pure Maple Syrup, + 2 Tablespoons

7. 1/4 cup Lard, (or coconut oil), + 2.5 Tablespoons, + 2 Tablespoons

8. 2 1/2 Tablespoons Beef, Great Lakes brand Unflavored Gelatin

9. 1 1/2 Tablespoon ground Cinnamon

10. 1/4 Tablespoon ground Cloves

11. 2 Tablespoons Raw Honey

Process

1. Preheat the oven to 325 degrees F and grease an 8- inch spring-form pan with either lard or coconut oil. Drain the dates, and place all of the ingredients in a

food processor and process for a minute, until a thick and sticky mixture forms. You may be able to do this in a high-powered blender using the tamper, but be sure to stop to scrape the sides and take breaks because it will be hard on the motor. Don't overmix here - you want the dates to be slightly chunky and not completely incorporated.

2. Transfer the mixture to the spring-form pan and spread evenly along the bottom with a spatula. Bake in the oven for 18-20 minutes, or until a knife

comes out clean when gently inserted. Set aside to cool.

3. Combine all of the filling ingredients, cold in a pot. Turn the heat on medium-low, and heat, stirring constantly, for 5-10 minutes. The mixture should liquefy and the gelatin should dissolve. If you still have some chunks after 10 minutes, transfer to a blender and blend for a few seconds to incorporate.

4. Pour into the spring-form pan over the gingersnap crust. Place in the refrigerator to set for at least 3 hours.

5. To make the frosting, combine all of the ingredients in a small bowl. A thick, spreadable frosting should form. If it is too runny, add more arrowroot, a teaspoon at a time until desired thickness is reached. The frosting will harden when placed in the refrigerator and soften at room temperature (although it shouldn't melt). When you are ready to frost your cake, you can either use a frosting kit or apply it to the top with a spatula.

Notes

Do not add fresh ginger to the filling ingredients - it has an enzyme that breaks down the gelatin and will cause the cake not to set properly. This cake freezes well - if you don't eat it all, don't be afraid to freeze a few slices for later!

Strawberry, Rose, and Coconut Milkshake

This treat fully embraces spring with its sweet, creaminess of the fresh coconut, the bright, fruity strawberry, and the floral, springy hint of rose.

Prep time: 10 minutes

Servings: 4

Ingredients

12. 2 cup Coconut Meat, freshly scooped from a Young Thai Coconut

13. 2 1/4 cup Coconut Water, freshly poured from a Young Thai Coconut

14. 1 cup Strawberries, fresh or frozen

15. 1 Tablespoons Rose Water, food grade

16. 1/2 cup Ice Cubes, optional-use only if using fresh strawberries

17. 1 whole Coconut Cream, optional-for topping

Process

1. Whip the coconut cream in a large bowl using a hand or stand mixer, until fluffy. Set aside.

2. Place the coconut meat and coconut water in a high powered blender, and blend on high, until smooth and creamy.

3. Add the frozen strawberries and rose water, and continue to blend until there are no lumps.

4. Pour the milkshake into glasses, top with the whipped coconut cream, and serve.

Pork Tenderloin w/ Peach Mint Sauce

Simple and flavorful, this Pork Tenderloin with Peach Mint Sauce is a winner for dinner! SCD and Paleo approved!

Prep time: 10 minutes

Cook time: 25 minutes

Servings: 4

Ingredients

18. 5 lb Pork Loin, fat trimmed
19. 2 whole Peaches, skinned removed, diced
20. 1 sprig Mint Leaves, chopped
21. 1/2 Tablespoon Lemon Juice

22. 1/4 Tablespoon ground Cinnamon

Process

1. Preheat oven to 400 degrees. Preheat pan on medium heat. Season pork tenderloin on each side with salt and pepper. When the pan is hot, sear each side of the tenderloin until brown. Once properly seared, remove from the pan and place into a baking dish. Place in the oven and bake for 25 mins, or until internal temperature reaches 150 degrees.

2. While tenderloin is cooking, dice the peaches. Add the peaches, mint, lemon juice and cinnamon in a small food processor and blend until smooth.

3. When the tenderloin is cooked, let rest for 5 minutes on a cutting board. Once rested, cut and serve with the sauce.

Instant Pot Beef Stock (Bone Broth)

We love using our Instant Pot for making quick, and delicious bone broth, or stock. Homemade stock is a nutritious base for soups, stews, sauces, or simply just to sip on for the health benefits.

Prep time: 1 hour

Cook time: 1 hour and 15 minutes

Servings: 10

Ingredients

23. 3-4 lb grass-fed Beef bones, roasted

24. 3 whole Carrots, cut in half

25. 4 whole Celery, ribs

26. 1 Onion, sliced in half

27. 2 cloves Garlic, smashed with a knive

28. 1 Bay Leaf

29. 1 Tablespoon Himalayan Pink Salt

30. 1 Tablespoons Apple Cider Vinegar

31. 1 Instant Pot

Process

1. Preheat your oven to bake at 420 degrees.

2. Place the beef bones in a glass baking sheet, and sprinkle with salt if desired.

3. Roast the bones for 30 minutes, flip them to their other side, and

then roast for another 20 minutes.

4. While the bones are roasting, prepare the vegetables for the broth.

5. Place the roasted bones into your Instant Pot, and then add the carrot, celery, onion, garlic, bay leaf, salt, and apple cider vinegar.

6. Fill the Instant Pot with filtered water until it reaches about an inch below the max fill line.

7. Place the lid on, and seal, and set to manual high pressure for 75 minutes.

8. Once the broth is finished, remove the large bones and vegetable pieces, and then strain the broth through a fine mesh strainer.

9. Pour the strained broth back into the Instant Pot, if using immediately after for soup, or allow to cool and freeze for future use.

Notes

This recipe makes 10 cups of broth. When using beef marrow bones, it's best to allow the broth to cool slightly, so that you can scoop the excess fat off of the top before making

soup.

Apple Pie

It took me a while to come up with a good apple pie recipe, because boy, am I picky! I like a thick, flaky crust paired with perfectly seasoned but not mushy filling. Was that possible with AIP ingredients? Turns out, with a couple of extra steps, it is totally possible to make a pie that satisfies those requirements, and one that is allergen-free to boot! Here I use the hot-water-pour-over method to pre-cook the apples ever so slightly. Like I said, I detest mushy pie, and this extra step at the beginning yields apples that are perfectly cooked, yet still a little firm and not soggy at all! Before you start this recipe, make sure you read through the instructions for sequence and give yourself enough time for the cooling/drying steps (they are important to making the pie come out properly!). I recommend melting the coconut oil to measure and then placing it in the refrigerator to harden, which can add some time if you forget. I also want to reiterate not to fuss with the crust too much–get it to the shape you want, and then leave it alone. The little bits of coconut oil are what create the flakiness in the crust, and if you over mix or fuss with the dough with your fingers your pie will lose this quality. I tested this on a bunch of non-Paleo/AIP family and friends and they all gave it a seal of approval, so you can serve it at your holiday meal with confidence!

Prep time: 1 minute

Cook time: 1 minute

Servings: 6

Ingredients

32. 5 whole Granny Smith Apple, peeled, quartered, cored, and sliced thinly

33. 1/2 cup Coconut Palm Sugar, + 2 Tablespoons

34. 1 Tablespoons ground Cinnamon

35. 1/4 Tablespoon Sea Salt, + 1/4 Tablespoon

36. 1 whole Lemon, juiced

37. 1 cup Arrowroot Flour

38. 1/2 cup Coconut Flour

39. 3/4 cup Organic Coconut Oil, cold

40. 1/2 cup Water, cold

Process

1. Preheat your oven to 350 degrees. If you haven't measured out your coconut oil and water and then placed them in the refrigerator to cool, do it now.

2. Place the apple slices in a large bowl. Fill a large pot with enough water to soak all of the apple slices, and bring it to a boil. When it is hot, pour the water into the bowl with the apples until they are just covered. Let them sit in the hot water for 8

minutes, and then place in a colander to drain and set aside while you make the crust.

3. To make the crust, combine the arrowroot, coconut flour, palm sugar, and sea salt in a medium bowl and stir to combine. Using a pastry cutter, butterknives, or your fingers, cut in the cold coconut oil until you have pea-sized lumps. Add the cold water, and mix gently. The mixture will be crumbly and not like regular dough--don't over mix!

4. Place the mixture into a 9-inch pie dish. Using your fingers,

spread it evenly across the bottoms and up the sides. Prick some holes in the bottom of the crust with a fork. Again, the dough will not behave like regular pie dough, and the less you handle it the more flaky it will come out. Bake for 15 minutes and then set aside while you make the filling.

5. Lay out a clean kitchen towel and pour the apple slices on it, blotting them dry. Combine the coconut palm sugar, cinnamon, and salt in a large bowl, and then add the dry apple slices and mix

gently. Pour the mixture into the crust, arranging the slices as needed.Sprinkle the pie with lemon juice and place in the oven to cook for 30-35 minutes, until the crust is golden brown.

6. Let cool for 10-15 minutes and then serve.

Miso Glazed Salmon

This Miso Glazed Salmon is a healthy, simple, and flavorful dish that even your kids will like!

Prep time: 10 minutes

Cook time: 20 minutes

Servings: 4

Ingredients

41. 16 oz Wild Caught Salmon Filet, 4 (4 ounce filets)

42. 1 Tablespoons Pure Maple Syrup

43. 2 Tablespoons Coconut Aminos

44. 2 Tablespoons Water, warm

Process

1. Preheat oven to 350 degrees

2. Add all ingredients except salmon to a sauce pan

3. Heat over medium heat, stirring frequently, until glaze is formed (5-7 minutes)

4. Place salmon filets on baking sheet lined with parchment paper

5. brush glaze onto fish

6. bake for 20 minutes or until fish flakes easily with a fork, pausing to reglaze every 5 minutes

7. garnish with green onions and sesame seeds

Carob Chip Bars

A decadent bar spiked with carob chips and topped with a thick layer of coconut whip cream! A lot easier to make than it looks.

Prep time: 10 minutes

Cook time: 40 minutes

Servings: 6

Ingredients

- 2 whole Plantain, peeled and chopped
- 1/2 cup Pumpkin Puree
- 2 Tablespoons Tigernut Flour
- 1/2 Tablespoon Baking Soda
- 3 Tablespoons Organic Coconut Butter
- 1/4 cup Organic Coconut Oil

- 2 Tablespoons Raw Honey

- 2 cup Coconut Milk, chilled, just the cream

Process

1. preheat oven to 350 deg

2. place all ingredients in bowl of food processor and blend until smooth, a couple minutes

3. pour into a greased loaf pan

4. stir in 1/2 c carob chips by hand

5. bake for 40-50 min (until inserted knife comes out clean)

6. meanwhile, whip coconut cream (i used my food processor)

7. once bars are done, cool on counter the in the fridge for a couple hours

8. frost with whip cream and rechill in fridge

Notes

The pumpkin adds a creaminess to the bar, but you can't taste any "pumpkin." This bar is not very sweet, which according to my taste buds right now is good. But feel free to pl ay around with the sweetener. I used unsweetened carob chips too.

Bison Stew

Prep time: 20 minutes

Cook time: 6 hours

Servings: 4

Ingredients

- 2 lb Bison Steak Medallions

- 1 Tablespoons Organic Coconut Oil

- 2 cup Celery, chopped

- 3 sprig Thyme

- 3 sprig fresh Rosemary

- 1 head Cauliflower, chopped

- 1 Yellow Onion, chopped

- 1 quart Beef Broth, reduced sodium

- 1/2 Tablespoon Salt, to taste (and black pepper, if not following AIP)

Process

1. In a cast iron skillet, brown bison stew meat on all sides in coconut oil.

2. Transfer seared bison meat into a large soup pot.

3. Place chopped onion and celery into the pot with the bison.

4. Pour beef broth over meat.

5. Season liberally with salt and pepper.

6. Place herbs, and celery greens into the pot, and turn burner onto medium heat.

7. Bring stew to a boil, stirring often.

8. Once stew comes to a boil, turn heat down to low, and cover with a lid.

9. Simmer stew for 6-8 hours, adding the

    chopped cauliflower for the last hour of

    cooking.

One Pot Steamed Garlic and Herb Scallops with Veggies

Steamed Scallops with Garlic, Herb, and veggies all cooked in ONE POT! Cooking Scallops can seem intimating for some, but this paleo friendly dish is ready in 10 minutes and is SUPER easy to make. A Healthy Light meal for one or more!

Prep time: 5 minutes

Cook time: 10 minutes

Servings: 2

Ingredients

- 1/3 cup Water, or broth

- 1 Tablespoons Extra Virgin Olive Oil

- 1 Tablespoons Lemon Juice

- 1 pinch Sea Salt

- 1/4 Tablespoon dried Basil

- 1/4 Tablespoon Onion Powder, or onion salt

- 1/4 Tablespoon Garlic, minced

- 6 oz Scallops, 1 serving (4-5 medium to large)

- 1 cup Kale, spinach, greens or favorite vegetables - chopped

- 2 Tablespoons Greek Salad Dressing (click for recipe) , Dressing of choice.

Process

1. Place water and dash salt in small pot. Place steamer on top. In a separate bowl, toss your scallops in a bit of your favorite dressing (maybe 1-2 Tablespoons) and then add in your seasoning. Boil your water then Place scallops and veggies on top of steamer. cover and steam with boiled water for 7-8 minutes or until scallops are opaque.

2. Remove from pot and place everything on plate. Add more seasoning and dash of lemon juice.

3. Scallops serve one but you can add more and make it serve two or more!

4. Check scallops and veggies around 7-8 minutes to see if they are done.

5. Scallops are done when they are opaque in center and easy to slice, not chewy. You really can't undercook them.

6. If you are using smaller scallops, they will probably cook faster, around 5-6 minutes steamed.

Roasted Rosemary Beets

Prep time: 10 minutes

Cook time: 5 minutes

Servings: 2

Ingredients

- 2 Tablespoons Extra Virgin Olive Oil

- 2 Tablespoons fresh Rosemary, chopped

- 3 Beets, chopped

- 1/2 Tablespoon Salt, (and black pepper,

  if not following AIP)

Process

1. Preheat the oven to roast at 400°F.

2. In a baking dish, toss beets in olive

   oil, salt, pepper, and rosemary.

3. Roast beets for 35 minutes, or until crispy on the outside and tender in the center.

Slow Cooker Squash & Ground Beef Curry

Ground beef and acorn squash simmer away in a spiced pumpkin curry sauce for a stick-to-your-ribs, comforting meal that's made in the slow cooker!

Prep time: 10 minutes

Cook time: 6 hours

Servings: 6

Ingredients

- 2 lb Ground Beef

- 1 whole Acorn Squash, cut into 1/2 inch cubes

- 13 1/2 oz Coconut Milk, (one can)

- 15 oz Pumpkin Puree, (one can)

- 1 1/2 cup Water

- 1 1/2 Tablespoons Ginger Root, peeled and diced

- 5 cloves Garlic

- 1 whole Lemon, quartered

- 1/2 Tablespoons Garlic Powder

- 1/2 Tablespoons Onion Powder

- 1/2 Tablespoons Turmeric Powder

- 1 Tablespoon dried Cilantro

- 1 Tablespoon dried Basil

- 1 Tablespoon dried Dill

- 1 Tablespoon ground Cinnamon

- 1/2 Tablespoon ground Ginger

- 1/4 Tablespoon ground Cloves

- 1/2 cup Cilantro, (optional) for topping

Process

1. Break up the ground beef into small pieces, as small as you can make them.

2. Add the ground beef and all other ingredients (except the fresh cilantro) to your slow cooker. Squeeze the lemons into the slow cooker before adding them.

3. Cover and cook on low for 4-6 hours or on high for 2-3 hours. If you're nearby, break up the chunks of ground beef halfway through the cooking time. If you're not, do so at the end.

4. Serve with cauliflower rice (you'll need about 1 1/2 - 2 cauliflower heads' worth

of rice) and topped with fresh cilantro (optional).

Sweet + Tangy Pork Lettuce Wraps

I love an Asian inspired dish once in a while and lettuce wraps have always been a favorite. The autoimmune protocol can make it a bit tricky to create an amazing sauce but I think you guys are really going to love this one. It's sweet and tangy and all around perfect! Don't let the number of ingredients scare you. I promise this is an easy, fast recipe that can be thrown together on a busy weeknight. I used pork but you can easily substitute chicken or turkey or even veggies if you want to make it meatless.

Prep time: 15 minutes

Cook time: 20 minutes

Servings: 8

Ingredients

- 1 head Iceburg Lettuce

- 1 whole Carrots, Small size head

- 1/4 head Red Cabbage, Small size head

- 1 whole Mango, Sliced

- 1/4 cup Mint Leaves, Chopped

- 1/4 cup Cilantro, Chopped

- 1/2 whole Red Onion, Chopped

- 1 pieces Ginger Root, 1 inch piece

- 1 clove Garlic, Finely chopped

- 2 Tablespoons Red Wine Vinegar

- 3 Tablespoons Raw Honey

- 4 Tablespoons Coconut Aminos

- 1/8 Tablespoon Sea Salt

- 1 Tablespoons Extra Virgin Olive Oil

- 1 Tablespoons Orange Juice

- 1 lb Ground Pork

Process

1. Wash iceberg lettuce and cut into quarters. Peel leaves off to create wraps. Set aside.

2. Wash mango and cut into cubes.

3. Peel and chop red onion. Set aside.

4. Peel and julienne or thinly slice carrot and set aside.

5. Wash and chop mint and set aside.

6. Wash and chop cilantro and set aside.

7. Peel and finely chop ginger and garlic clove and set aside.

8. In a separate bowl add honey and warm just until it becomes a liquid. Add vinegar, coconut aminos, sea salt, ginger, garlic and orange juice. Mix well to combine. Set sauce aside.

9. In a skillet add olive oil and meat. Break up meat and stir continually until it is half cooked. This should take about 5-10 min.

10. Add onions and cook an additional 5 min. Stir every minute or so.

11. Add sauce, mix well and cook another 5-10 min or until meat is browned and sauce starts to thicken. Stir every few minutes.

12. To serve place a spoonful of pork on top of a lettuce leaf and top with cabbage, carrot, cilantro, mint and mango.

Pizette

Prep time: 25 minutes

Cook time: 25 minutes

Servings: 4

Ingredients

- 1/3 cup Coconut Flour, (crust)

- 1/3 cup Arrowroot Powder, (crust)

- 1/3 cup Tapioca Starch, (crust)

- 1 Tablespoons Beef, Great Lakes brand Unflavored Gelatin, (crust)

- 6 Tablespoons Lard, (crust) at room temperature, soft but not melted

- 1/2 cup Water, (crust)

- 1 Tablespoon Salt, (crust)

- 1/4 lb Uncured Pepperoni, (filling)

- 2 Tablespoons fresh Basil, (filling) chopped

- 1 cup Caulifredo Sauce

Process

1. [For the crust] Mix together dry ingredients (coconut, tapioca and arrowroot flours, gelatin, and salt).

2. Blend in lard using a fork or pastry blender.

3. Mix water in, stirring until a ball of dough forms.

4. Wet your hands, then place the ball of dough on a parchment-lined pizza stone.

5. Flatten the dough with your palms, then place another sheet of parchment over the top.

6. Using a rolling pin, flatten the dough into a big circle.

7. Roll out to about 1/4" thickness. You can use your hand to run a little more water around the edges if it threatens to crack.

8. Remove top parchment and prepare the fillings.

9. [For the filling] Spread sauce over crust, leaving 2-3 inches bare on edges.

10. Top with meat, basil and any additional toppings of choice.

11. Using the parchment paper underneath, carefully fold up the edges of the crust over the edge of the fillings, again spreading a little water over the crust if need be.

12. Cook at 425 for 25 minutes.

Tempura Shrimp

This light and crispy batter is perfect for any type of fried seafood (just check out our Fish 'n Chips recipe!) While it takes a little finesse and patience, the result is SO worth it! Serves 4 as a main dish, or 8 as an appetizer.

Prep time: 30 minutes

Cook time: 40 minutes

Servings: 2

Ingredients

- 3/4 cup Arrowroot Flour

- 1/4 cup Cassava Flour, plus 2 tablespoons

- 2 Tablespoon Baking Powder

- 1/8 Tablespoon ground Ginger

- 1/2 Tablespoon Himalayan Pink Salt

- 1/8 Tablespoon Fish Sauce, about 3 drops

- 1 cup Sparkling Water

- 2 Tablespoons Coconut Aminos

- Organic Coconut Oil, Tropical Traditions steam refined coconut oil. Aim for at least 2 inches of oil in pot

- 2 lb Raw Shrimp, wild caught, tail on

Process

1. Whisk together the dry ingredients in a large mixing bowl; only adding the 1/4 of cassava to start.

2. Pour in the fish sauce, coconut aminos, and sparkling water while whisking to combine. If batter is too loose, add a tablespoon of cassava at a time until the batter is about as thick as pancake batter (it should coat the whisk).

3. Choose a pot with high walls and a small diameter to maximize oil depth for frying. Add enough coconut oil (or lard, or your choice of cooking fat) to have a minimum depth of 3" of oil. Heat to 320 degrees Fahrenheit, monitoring the temperature with a candy thermometer.

4. Clean and peel the shrimp, removing all shell and only leaving the tail on. De-vein the shrimp.

5. Prepare a wire rack over a cookie sheet to allow fried shrimp to drain.

6. Dip the shrimp in the batter to coat, one at a time. Slowly lower into the hot oil, holding the shrimp by the tail, and allowing the batter to being to fry

before releasing the shrimp. This will prevent the shrimp from sticking to the pot.

7. Working with only 2-3 shrimp in the pot at a time, cook the shrimp for about 3 minutes, until the batter is golden brown. Place on a wire rack to drain. Repeat until all shrimp are fried.

Autoimmune Paleo Orange Teriyaki Meatballs

What makes these so fantastic, is the strategic placement of spices. Orange zest and diced green onions in the meatballs. A sauce driven with fresh orange juice, fresh ginger and coconut aminos. It is an extremely well balanced dish. The sauce is wonderfully concentrated, but for 2 pounds of chicken is plenty.

Prep time: 20 minutes

Cook time: 25 minutes

Servings: 4

Ingredients

- 2 lb boneless skinless Chicken Breasts, Ground

- 1/2 cup Green Onion, chopped

- 2 Tablespoons Orange Zest

- 2/3 cup Orange Juice, fresh

- 2 Tablespoon Ginger Root, minced

- 1/4 cup Coconut Aminos

- 1 Tablespoons Apple Cider Vinegar

- 1 clove Garlic, minced

- 1 Tablespoons Raw Honey

Process

1. In a bowl, mix ground chicken (you can use any kind; breast or a blend) orange zest, pinch salt and green onions. On a

parchment lined cookie sheet, form 2 1/2 inch sized meatballs. Bake at 350 until internal temperature reaches 170 degrees. Mine took about 30 minutes.

2. In a saucepan, add coconut aminos grated ginger, garlic, honey, vinegar and fresh orange juice. Bring to a simmer and reduce until sauce coats the back of a spoon. It will simmer for about 10 minutes and then start to watch it closely. It will start to foam and bubble as it is reducing and almost ready. You want the sauce to be the consistency of maple syrup.

3. When meatballs are cooked, place in a

    bowl and drizzle with the sauce. Gently

    toss to coat all the meatballs.

AIP Blackberry Cobbler

Here is a delicious blackberry cobbler recipe. It's ready to eat in under an hour, filled with healthy berries, and is a cinch to throw together.

Prep time: 15 minutes

Cook time: 35 minutes

Servings: 6

Ingredients

- 12 oz Blackberries

- 2 Tablespoons Organic Coconut Oil, plus more for greasing

- 3 Tablespoons Water

- 1/4 cup Arrowroot Flour

- 1/4 cup Coconut Flour

- 1/4 cup Raw Honey

- 1/4 Tablespoon Salt

- 3/4 Tablespoon Baking Soda

- 1 1/4 Tablespoon Lemon Juice

Process

1. Preheat oven to 300. Lightly grease an 8×8 baking dish with coconut oil.

2. Spread blackberries evenly in bottom of pan.

3. Mix remaining ingredients on medium speed until combined. Spread over blackberries.

4. Bake for 35-40 minutes, until entire top is golden brown.

Warm Shrimp Salad with Bok Choy

Bok choy is a vegetable that pairs well with Asian-inspired flavors. Here, we've combined bok choy, shrimp, and sesame dressing. The result is a dish which is presented as a salad, but brings together all the flavors associated with a stir-fry.

Prep time: 5 minutes

Cook time: 10 minutes

Servings: 4

Ingredients

- 1 head large Bok Choy

- 1/3 lb Raw Shrimp

- 1/4 Tablespoon Fish Sauce

- 3 Tablespoons Coconut Aminos

- 2 clove Garlic

- 1/4 cup Watercress

Process

1. Heat a large skillet over medium-high heat.

2. Rinse the bok choy, and remove the large white veins near the bottom of each leaf. Chop the leaves lengthwise, and set aside.

3. Place the shrimp in the skillet, and stir in the fish sauce and coconut aminos. Sauté for 4-5 minutes.

4. Add the minced garlic and watercress, and continue to sauté until the shrimp is completely opaque.

5. Add the bok choy, and sauté 1-2 minutes, until it begins to soften slightly.

6. Remove the skillet from the heat, and serve immediately.

Beets and Sweets Hash

I have to be totally honest I got this idea for Beets and Sweets from a vegetable chip company that you can find in super markets. I mean I would totally buy them if they weren't fried in vegetable oils, it is probably a good thing they are though because I would be eating them by the bag full...everyday. I have no self control. Well I figured why not incorporate two healthy vegetables into a side-dish and add bacon. So easy and so delicious!

Prep time: 10 minutes

Cook time: 45 minutes

Servings: 4

Ingredients

- 1 whole Sweet Potato, peeled and cubed to 1/4" pieces
- 1 whole Beets, peeled and cubed to 1/4" pieces
- 2 Tablespoons Extra Virgin Olive Oil

- 3 pieces Bacon, chopped

- 2 whole Green Onion, chopped

Process

1. preheat oven to 375F

2. coat potato and beet cubes with olive oil, salt and pepper

3. roast for 35-40 minutes until fork tender

4. dice bacon and cook until crispy, drain fat reserving 1T

5. add beets and sweets to the pan and heat together with bacon and reserved bacon fat

6. garnish with chopped scallions and serve

Turkey Breakfast Sausage

Two ingredients = easiest recipe ever (if you can even call it a recipe!) Whip this up with any type of ground meat (beef, chicken, pork), form into patties, and cook them up in a skillet. Breakfast, solved.

Prep time: 2 minutes

Cook time: 10 minutes

Servings: 4

Ingredients

- 1 lb Ground Turkey
- 1 Tablespoons Primal Palate Breakfast Blend
- 1/2 Tablespoons Lard

Process

1. Mix the ground turkey and spice blend in a bowl thoroughly. Form into patties by dividing the mixture in half, then in half again, and all portions in half one last time (giving you 8 small patties).

2. Heat the lard, or you choice of cooking fat, over medium heat in a skillet. Fry the patties about 4-5 minutes on each side, until fully cooked (may take 10 minutes, or longer, depending on the thickness.)

3. Serve alongside your favorite breakfast dishes!

AIP Starch-Free Coconut Cream Pie

Paleo and non-paleo alike, You can take this to parties and get-togethers without a single person ever guessing it's a healthy version. Note: This does not take 4 hours to make, it just has to chill for four hours.

Prep time: 30 minutes

Cook time: 15 minutes

Servings: 8

Ingredients

- 1/2 cup Coconut Flour, (for the crust)

- 1/4 Tablespoon Salt, (for the crust)

- 1/4 Tablespoon Baking Soda, (for the crust)

- 3/4 Tablespoon ground Cinnamon, (for the crust)

- 1/3 cup Organic Coconut Oil, melted (for the crust)

- 1/2 Tablespoon Pure Vanilla Extract, (for the crust)

- 1/3 cup Raw Honey, (for the filling)

- 2 Tablespoon Unflavored, Knox brand Gelatin, (for the filling)

- 1 cup shredded Coconut, toasted at 350 for 5-6 minutes (for the filling)

- 16 oz Coconut Milk, (for the filling)

- 1/2 cup Organic Coconut Butter, (for the filling)

- 1 1/2 Tablespoon Vanilla Extract, (for the filling)

- 1/4 Tablespoon Sea Salt, (for the filling)

Process

1. [For the crust] Preheat oven to 350.

2. In small bowl, whisk together dry ingredients: coconut flour, salt, baking soda and cinnamon. Set aside.

3. In stand mixer, beat wet ingredients together on medium.

4. Add dry ingredients, mixing until fully combined.

5. Scrape dough into 9" pie plate. Place a piece of parchment paper (large enough to cover entire pie plate) over the crust. Using small hand-held rolling pin (or use a small drinking glass turned on its

side), roll crust flat to cover the bottom and sides of the pie plate. The dough will thicken as the gelatin sets, so this may take some extra rolling compared to an egg-based crust.

6. Bake for 10-12 minutes, until golden brown. While crust is baking, toast coconut and prepare pie filling.

7. [For the filling] Toast coconut on a baking sheet for 5-6 minutes, until golden brown (Do not skip this step. Without it, the pie will be colorless and semi-translucent. It also adds great toasty flavor!)

8. In medium saucepan over medium heat, Whisk all ingredients together, except for the gelatin and toasted coconut.

9. Scoop out 2 teaspoons of the milk mixture and place it into a small dish. Add the gelatin and let it absorb the milk to create a rubbery mixture.

10. Cover the milk mixture and bring to a simmer. Whisk in rubbery gelatin mixture and whisk vigorously until the gelatin is completely dissolved. Turn off heat.

11. Stir in the coconut, and pour the mixture into the prepared graham pie crust.

12. Refrigerate for 4 hours, until completely

cool and hardened throughout.

Slow Cooker Ham

A flavorful dish that you can just toss in the crockpot and forget about! Both Paleo and Autoimmune Paleo friendly.

Prep time: 5 minutes

Cook time: 4 minutes

Servings: 8

Ingredients

- 4 - 6 lb Ham

- 1/4 cup Raw Honey

- 1/2 cup Orange Juice

- 2 Tablespoon dried Rosemary

- 4 Tablespoons Organic Coconut Oil

- 1 Tablespoon Orange Zest

- 1 Tablespoons Apple Cider Vinegar

Process

1. Place ham in slow cooker.

2. Put the rest of the ingredients on the ham.

3. Cook on low for 4-6 hours.

Notes

You can use a spiral sliced ham for this but I'd keep the cooking time more on the low end (closer to 4 hours or even less) as the slices allow it to cook faster and get dried out faster.

A creamy, grain-free and dairy-free hot breakfast cereal made with caramelized cauliflower! It's healthy, comforting, and delicious!

Prep time: 10 minutes

Cook time: 40 minutes

Servings: 4

Ingredients

- 1 head Cauliflower, broken into 1-inch florets

- 4 Tablespoons Organic Coconut Oil, divided

- 3 Tablespoons Coconut Milk

- 2 Tablespoons Coconut Palm Sugar

- 2 Tablespoons Pure Maple Syrup, plus more for drizzling (optional)

- 1/4 Tablespoon Sea Salt, heaping

- 1/4 Tablespoon ground Cinnamon, plus more for sprinkling (optional)

- 1 pinch ground Cloves

Process

1. Preheat the oven to 425 degrees F. Line a large baking sheet with foil.

2. In a large, microwave-safe bowl, heat 2 tablespoons of coconut oil in the microwave until it's melted. Add the cauliflower florets and drizzle over 2 tablespoons of melted coconut oil. Toss

the cauliflower florets and toss with your hands or a large spoon until the cauliflower is completely coated with oil.

3. Lay the florets in a single, even layer on the baking sheet. Place the baking sheet in the oven and roast the cauliflower for 20-25 minutes or until tender and the edges are turning a deep brown.

4. Remove the baking sheet from the oven and add the roasted cauliflower, 2 tablespoons coconut oil, coconut milk, sugar, maple syrup, salt, cinnamon, and cloves to the bowl of a large food processor. Process on high for 3 minutes, or until the mixture is thick, creamy, and blended.

5. Spoon into bowls, top with cinnamon
   and maple syrup and/or fresh fruit
   (optional) and enjoy!

Sea Salt & Lime Spinach Chips

A delicious, wholesome version of those super addictive (and super terrible for you) lime tortilla chips!

Prep time: 5 minutes

Cook time: 30 minutes

Servings: 6

Ingredients

- 1 whole Lime, about 1 1/2 Tablespoons zest + 2 Tablespoon juice, divided

- 1/2 Tablespoon Sea Salt

- 8 cup Spinach, whole leaves, measured packed

- 2 Tablespoons Extra Virgin Olive Oil

Process

1. Preheat the oven to 275F. Line 2 baking sheets with nonstick pads, or lightly grease them.

2. In a small bowl, use your fingers to rub together the zest and the salt.

3. In a large mixing bowl, toss the spinach with the olive oil to thoroughly coat. Then add the lime salt and toss again to distribute a little bit of the salt on each leaf. Use your hands if necessary.

4. Distribute the spinach between the two prepared cookie sheets in an even layer (do not crowd the leaves). Sprinkle each batch with a teaspoon of lime juice.

5. Bake for 30-35 minutes (you may need less time depending on how fresh your spinach is, so keep an eye on it) until the leaves are withered and very thin.

6. Remove from oven, and let the chips cool completely on the pan before serving.

Notes

You have to use large spinach leaves, not baby spinach, for this recipe. It is best to eat these chips as soon as they've cooled. If you need to store them, the best way is in an open container in the fridge. If you cover them, they'll get soggy though. Even uncovered, they will lose some of their crispness overnight.

Festive Green Spritzer

Last year I spent some time researching juicers because I wanted to incorporate juices in to my diet. After much time researching I finally decided on one. I picked up some veggies on the way home and then immediately started making a drink. I was used to drinking them and really didn't think much about how "green" it tasted. Some people need to get used to drinking greens in a juice. It got me thinking a lot about ways to use my juicer to make juices for people who weren't used to them and also for entertaining. I wanted people to see that healthy foods can be fun and festive too! This juice recipe is really inspired by things I have been getting from the farmer's market lately and also inspired by bold fall flavors. It is a great blend of sweet, tangy, and spicy. All the flavors really balance each other and you don't get an overwhelming kale taste for those who maybe don't like the flavor as much. Topping the juice with some club soda not only gives the juice a festive spritz but also leaves a very refreshing taste on your pallet! Feel free to adjust anything according to taste!

Prep time: 5 minutes

Servings: 2

Ingredients

- 1 whole Cucumber, medium
- 1 whole Lemon, large
- 3 whole Bartlett Pear

- 3 whole Kale, large leaves

- 1 oz Ginger Root, three inch piece

- 16 oz Sparkling Water

Process

1. Peel some of the rind off the lemon and core the pears.

2. Put the cucumber, lemon, pears, kale, and ginger through the juicer.

3. Pour the mixture through a fine mesh sieve. Fill a tall glass with ice and add about one cup of juice concentrate.

4. Top with about u00bd cup of club soda and enjoy! Adjust club soda and juice to taste.

Notes

I have weight measurements on the blog if you wish to use exact measurements. All of these ingredients can be changed according to taste. If you want it sweeter then add more Pear. Add more lemon for tartness and more ginger for spice!

AIP Breadsticks

These little babies are absolutely delicious. The first time I made them my (non-paleo) husband said, "Wow! These actually taste like real bread!" And the best part of this recipe? They are super quick and easy. In fact, you could whip these up every night of the week if you wanted to!

Prep time: 10 minutes

Cook time: 10 minutes

Servings: 8

Ingredients

- 4 Tablespoons Extra Virgin Olive Oil, divided (3 Tablespoons for breadsticks, 1 Tablespoons for topping)
- 3 Tablespoons Water
- 1/3 cup Arrowroot Flour
- 1/3 cup Coconut Flour
- 1/2 Tablespoon Baking Soda
- 1 Tablespoon dried Rosemary
- 1 1/2 Tablespoon Lemon Juice
- 1 Tablespoons Beef, Great Lakes brand Unflavored Gelatin, plus 3 TABLESPOONS water (to create egg substitute)
- 1/8 Tablespoon Garlic Powder, for topping

- 1/8 Tablespoon Sea Salt, for topping

Process

1. Preheat oven to 350.

2. In standing mixer, place all ingredients except for gelatin egg substitute.

3. Prepare gelatin egg: Mix 1 tablespoon gelatin into 1 tablespoon cool water. Add 2 tablespoons of boiling water and whisk vigorously until completely dissolved and frothy. Add to mixing bowl and combine on medium until a thick dough forms.

4. Scrape dough onto sheet of parchment paper. Divide dough into 8 balls. Grease hands with olive oil and roll each ball into 8" sticks. If dough cracks, wet your fingertips to add a bit more moisture.

5. Brush breadsticks evenly with olive oil. Sprinkle garlic and sea salt over top.

6. Bake 10-12 minutes, until tops are golden brown.

Cauliflower Rice

Prep time: 10 minutes

Cook time: 7 minutes to 9 minutes

Servings: 4

Ingredients

- 1 clove Garlic, minced

- 1 Tablespoons Organic Coconut Oil

- 1 head Cauliflower

- 1/2 cup Yellow Onion, chopped

- 1/2 Tablespoon Himalayan Pink Salt, to taste (and black pepper, if not following AIP)

- 1 Tablespoon Primal Palate Garlic & Herb Seasoning, (sub: 1/2 Tablespoon himalayan pink salt)

Process

1. Rinse cauliflower under cool water and pat dry.

2. Using a cheese grater, grate the cauliflower to a coarse texture (approximately the size of rice grains). Using a food processor to pulse the cauliflower to desired texture works as well.

3. Heat the coconut oil in a skillet over medium heat.

4. Sauté the onion and garlic for 3–4 minutes, or until the onion is relatively translucent.

5. Add in the cauliflower rice and
   continue to sauté for 4–5
   minutes.

6. Season with salt and pepper, and
   serve.

www.ingramcontent.com/pod-product-compliance
Lightning Source LLC
Chambersburg PA
CBHW071517150726
48000CB00002B/581